# A COMPREHENSIVE GUIDE TO JUDO

## Mastering The Techniques, Training, And Tactics Of Judo

**RANDY AMOS**

# Contents

# CHAPTER ONE
## Judo: A Brief Overview

The combat sport and martial art known as judo has its roots in Japan, in the latter half of the nineteenth century. Jigoro Kano created this style of grappling, throwing, and joint locking techniques to control one's opponent.

Millions of people all around the world participate in judo, both as a sport and a form of exercise. Since the 1964 Summer Olympics, it has also been an Olympic sport.

Judo is founded on the ideals of mutual benefit and efficiency. Its methods are based on the idea that a smaller, weaker opponent can be defeated by employing leverage and timing to their advantage. Judo is well-known for its positive effects on health and wellness, self-control, and social graces.

This primer on Judo will cover the fundamentals of the sport, including its origins, philosophy, and rules. Judo is a one-of-a-kind and fulfilling experience that can aid in the growth of one's physical and mental abilities, as well as one's character and values, whether one is a novice or a seasoned practitioner.

## The Origins And Development Of Judo

Jigoro Kano, a Japanese martial artist, established judo in Tokyo in 1882. Kano, a proficient practitioner of multiple forms of ancient Japanese martial arts, set out to design a methodology that would be more suited for self-defense, as well as for use in the classroom and as a means of personal growth.

Jujitsu was just one of the many martial systems from which Kano drew inspiration while creating his own style, which he termed Judo. Instead of depending on attacks or physical strength, he advocated for the use of throws and leverage to overpower opponents.

He also added a code of ethics and a set of training procedures that emphasized self-control and consideration for others.

Judo's popularity in Japan skyrocketed, prompting Kano to establish the Kodokan as a training facility and advocacy group.

Kano traveled extensively to promote Judo and build Judo clubs and organizations around the world, with the Kodokan emerging as the sport's epicenter.

There has been an Olympic competition in judo ever since the sport was featured in the Summer Games in 1964. Judo, one of the most popular martial arts and combat sports in the world, is governed internationally by the International Judo Federation (IJF), which was founded in 1951.

New methods and strategies in judo have been developed and polished by athletes and instructors over the years. Maximum efficiency, mutual welfare and benefit, and respect for others are only few of Judo's enduring core ideals that have guided the sport from its inception.

## Throws And Fundamental Moves

Judo is a type of martial art that emphasizes throwing, locking joints, and grappling. Some of the most frequent Judo throws and techniques are described below.

• Using a circular motion of the foot, the opponent's leg is swept out from under them in the throwing technique known as Osoto-gari (Major Outer Reap).

• To perform a Seoi-nage (Shoulder Throw), the practitioner throws the opponent over his or her shoulder.

• In the grappling technique known as kesa-gatame (Scarf Hold), one person pins the other person to the ground by wrapping an arm around the opponent's neck.

• By bending their arm in the opposite direction, practitioners of the joint lock technique known as ude-garami (arm lock) render their opponent's arm immobile.

• Sweeping the opponent's leg with the hip and then throwing them over is the harai-goshi (sweeping hip throw) method.

• The Juji-gatame (Cross Arm Lock) is a joint lock in which the practitioner applies pressure to the elbow joint to paralyze the opponent's arm.

• In the throwing technique known as Ouchi-gari (Major Inner Reap), the opponent's leg is swept out from under them in a scissor-like action.

• Kata-guruma (Shoulder Wheel) is a type of throwing maneuver in which the attacker is lifted onto their back and then thrown after being rotated in a circle.

The techniques and throws shown here are only a small sample of what Judo has to offer. Judoka must be proficient in a wide range of techniques and know how to properly employ them.

# CHAPTER TWO
## Tools And Jargon Of Judo

Judo, a form of martial art from Japan, places an emphasis on ground fighting and submission holds. Judo utilizes the following tools and jargon most frequently:

**Equipment:**

• The judo gi consists of a jacket and pants made of thick cotton and is worn by practitioners.

• Belt – The belt is used to fasten the jacket and also serves as a status symbol.

• Judo takes place on a special mat called a tatami, which is used for both practice and competition.

•The kata demonstration wooden sword, or shinai.

**Terminology:**

• Sensei is a Japanese title for professor or tutor.

• Dojo means "martial arts school" in Japanese.

• Ukemi is the art of falling with the least amount of harm possible.

• During randori, practitioners engage in free-form sparring.

• Kata refers to a set sequence of techniques that have been choreographed ahead of time.

• Ippon is the highest possible score in judo and is given for a perfectly executed throw that results in the opponent landing on their back.

• Waza are the many judo techniques and maneuvers, including throws and submissions.

• Uke refers to the target of a technique or maneuver.

• Tori is the one carrying out the action.

• Kesa Gatame is an armlock in which the tori encircles the uke's neck and traps the uke's arm.

• Osoto gari is a sweeping throw in which the tori sweeps the uke's leg with his or her own leg, bringing the uke to the ground.

• The tori seoi nages the uke over their hip by lifting them onto their shoulder and then throwing them.

• The tori uses his or her legs to capture and hyperextend the uke's arm in a juji gatame.

Just a few examples of judo terminology and gear are included above. Learning the techniques and becoming skilled in the sport requires time and effort, just like any other form of martial arts.

## Variety In Judo

Judo, a combat sport and martial art from Japan, is based on throwing and grappling techniques. The following are some Judo techniques:

• Judo's founding father, Jigoro Kano, created the Kodokan style in the 19th century. The ideas of mutual benefit and efficient use of resources are emphasized.

• Kosen Judo is a subset of Judo that originated in early 20th-century Japanese academies. When compared to Kodokan Judo, this style prioritizes battling on the ground and submitting your opponent.

• Freestyle Judo is an offshoot of traditional Judo that originated in the United States during the 1960s. When compared to conventional

Judo, it is more relaxed and permits a broader range of techniques.

• It is believed that Brazilian Jiu-Jitsu evolved from Judo in the early 20th century. It incorporates techniques from other martial arts and places greater emphasis on ground fights and submissions than Judo.

• Sambo is a form of Russian martial arts that emerged at the turn of the twentieth century. It incorporates striking skills into a synthesis of Judo and wrestling.

• This style of Judo, known as "Judo for Self-Defense," places an emphasis on techniques that can be employed in legitimate self-defense scenarios. It could involve methods that are forbidden in official Judo competitions.

Judo as a whole is a flexible martial art with a wide variety of schools of thought from which students can select the one that best matches their needs.

# CHAPTER THREE
## Learn The Art Of Judo

**Judo instruction typically consists of the following:**

• Ukemi means "the art of graceful falling." Learning how to fall safely is a crucial aspect of training for the judo techniques that entail throwing or taking down an opponent.

• Nage-waza means "throwing techniques" in Japanese. Judoka learn how to throw with various techniques and perfect their form and timing.

• Grappling techniques, such as pins, chokes, and joint locks, are collectively known as katame-waza. Students learn both how to properly employ these strategies and how to avoid them in the future.

• Randori is a term for impromptu sparring between two practitioners. Students apply their skills in a more fluid, unexpected environment, where they must anticipate and respond to their opponent's actions.

• Shiai means "in competition" in Judo. To score points and ultimately win the match, competitors attempt to throw or pin their opponent.

• Judo training also incorporates physical conditioning, including exercises to build strength, stamina, and flexibility. • Meditation and other forms of mental exercise like visualisation may also play a role.

Dojos, or training halls, are common places for judokas to hone their skills under the watchful eye of knowledgeable instructors. It is common practice for novices to begin with fundamentals and graduate to more complex methods as they gain competence.

## Methods Of Training In Judo

Judo is a martial art that calls for stamina, quickness, and adaptability from its practitioners. In order to better your Judo, try these workouts and exercises:

• Judo requires a great deal of speed and explosiveness, so it is crucial to strengthen your cardiovascular system to withstand these demands. Stamina can be increased through cardiovascular exercise like jogging, cycling, or swimming.

• Plyometrics are a type of workout that emphasizes explosive movements and has been shown to increase both power and speed. Jump squats, box jumps, and explosive push-ups are just a few examples.

• Training your upper body, core, and legs to increase strength will help you perform Judo techniques with more force and precision. Strength training includes activities like squatting, deadlifting, pulling, and pushing.

• Incorporating agility activities like ladder drills or cone drills into your workouts can be helpful because judo requires rapid footwork and agility.

• Judo requires a great deal of twisting and turning of the body, therefore flexibility training is crucial. Flexibility can be boosted by the practice of yoga or other forms of dynamic stretching.

• Drilling your Judo techniques over and over can help you learn them by heart and make your movements feel more natural. Grappling dummies and practice sessions with a training partner are great ways to hone your skills.

• Because of the emphasis on grasping in judo, it is vital to train certain muscles. Using a grip trainer or simply hanging from a bar are two great ways to increase your grip strength.

Please warm up before beginning any fitness routine and get expert advice if you have any questions. The best way to get better at Judo is to train and practice often.

# CHAPTER FOUR
## Judo As A Sport And A Means Of Defense

The Japanese martial art of judo centers on taking down an opponent through throws and grappling. While competition and self-defense use very similar strategies, there are subtle but important distinctions in execution.

To gain points in Judo, competitors attempt to pin or throw their opponents to the ground. To win a match, you either need to score more points than your opponent or throw them so hard that they can not get up. Judo is a sport that is conducted under strict rules and regulations and in a regulated setting during competition.

Judo techniques can be used to restrain an assailant and keep yourself safe in a dangerous circumstance. But in self-defense, the goal is not to win, it is to stop the threat as soon and as easily as possible. There are no referees or rules to rely on when you are in a self-defense situation, and the scene is generally chaotic.

Judokas must learn to modify their strategies according to the conditions they face. Throws may need to be adjusted for uneven ground, and strategies may need to be reworked to deal with several attackers.

Overall, the Judo techniques used for competition and self-defense are very similar, although their focus and application can vary greatly. The aim of competition is to rack up points and win matches, but the goal of self-defense is to eliminate danger as soon and effectively as possible.

# The Core Values And Ideals Of Judo

Like other forms of martial art, judo is founded on a guiding philosophy and set of principles. Some fundamental tenets of Judo are as follows:

• Judo's basic premise of mutual welfare and benefit states that its practice is beneficial to both the practitioner and society at large. According to this tenet, Judo training should encourage its participants to treat one another with dignity and work together toward a common goal.

- The maxim of "maximum efficiency, minimum effort" stresses the need of performing Judo moves with as little effort as possible. This guiding philosophy emphasizes smarts over brawn.

- This philosophy, known as Seiryoku Zenyo, Jita Kyoei, emphasizes the need of working together for the greater good in order to make the best possible use of energy.

- Ju: This fundamental concept of Judo means "gentleness" or "flexibility." It stresses the importance of only resorting to physical force when all other options have been exhausted. Instead, Judokas should concentrate on using their opponents' own strength and speed against them.

• In Judo, technique and form are honed via the practice of Kata, which are structured sequences of motion. They assist build muscle memory and technique, with an emphasis on the core judo principles.

• Randori: Randori is free practice, where students can put their newly acquired skills to use in a more natural and unstructured environment. It stresses the value of flexibility and quick thinking in the face of uncertainty.

In a nutshell, Judo's guiding principles and philosophy stress the value of friendship and teamwork, the wise application of energy, and the primacy of skill and flexibility above physical might.

## Modern Judo And Society

The Japanese martial art of judo, which was developed towards the end of the 19th century, has had a profound effect on contemporary society. Some of the ways in which

Judo has impacted contemporary society are listed below.

• Judo has been an Olympic sport since 1964, and its competitions often draw large crowds. Yasuhiro Yamashita, David Douillet, and Teddy Riner are just a few of the famous athletes who hail from this region.

• The principals of Judo, which include turning an opponent's strength against them, have been adopted by a wide variety of different martial arts and self-defense methods.

• Judo's philosophical underpinnings stress the value of humility, self-control, and continuous growth. Many professionals, even those who do not compete, now follow these guidelines.

• Many works of popular culture, including films and television episodes, have included judo as a plot element. You Only Live Twice, starring Sean Connery as James Bond, includes a scene in which Bond employs Judo to fend off many assailants.

• Judo is a terrific method to work on your strength, flexibility, and endurance, all of which contribute to a healthy body and mind. Discipline and focus necessary in training can lead to decreased stress and enhanced self-confidence, both of which contribute to better mental health.

Both as a sport and a philosophy, Judo has made major contributions to contemporary society. Many people found inspiration in its emphasis on discipline, respect, and self-improvement, and its influence can be observed in many facets of contemporary life.

## Conclusion

Judo is a martial art that has significantly influenced contemporary society. It is more than just a way of life that preaches humility, self-control, and dedication to one's craft.

Many people throughout the world have taken up judo as a way to get in shape, discover new skills, and strengthen their minds. Its ideas have been adopted by a wide variety of martial arts and self-defense systems, and it has even made its way into fiction. Judo is a great sport to try out whether your goal is to compete at the top levels or you are just looking for a new way to get in shape.

**THE END**

www.ingramcontent.com/pod-product-compliance
Lightning Source LLC
Chambersburg PA
CBHW061740250726

48657CB00002B/1027